LOW RESIDUE DIET

A Comprehensive Guide to Digestive Health and Symptom Relief

Adams .U. Morris

TABLE OF CONTENTS

Chapter 1 5

Introduction to Low Residue Diet 5

Chapter 2 17

Understanding Residue and Its Impact........17

Chapter 3 29

Benefits and Risks of a Low Residue Diet.....29

Chapter 4 45

Foods to Avoid on a Low Residue Diet.........45

Chapter 5 59

Low Residue Diet Meal Planning..................59

Chapter 6 75

Nutritional Considerations on a Low Residue Diet 75

Chapter 7 92

Practical Strategies for Success on a Low Residue Diet...92

Chapter 8 108

Long-Term Management and Beyond: Life After a Low Residue Diet............................108

conclusion 123

CHAPTER 1

Introduction to Low Residue Diet

In the world of nutrition and dietary choices, the term "low residue diet" may sound a bit unfamiliar to many. However, it's a dietary approach that can have a significant impact on our digestive health, and this chapter serves as our gateway to understanding its fundamentals.

Let's start with the basic question: What is a low residue diet?

In simple terms, a low residue diet is a specialized eating plan designed to reduce the amount of undigested food and fiber that remains in the colon after digestion. This may leave you wondering why we would want to reduce residue in our diet in the first place. To answer that, we need to delve into the intricacies of our digestive system.

Understanding Digestion and Residue

Digestion is the process by which our body breaks down the foods we eat into smaller, absorbable components, primarily in the small intestine. What's left after this process, and what eventually reaches the colon, is referred to as "residue." This residue consists of indigestible components, such as fiber, as well as waste products.

The colon, also known as the large intestine, plays a crucial role in absorbing water and electrolytes from the residue, forming stool, and eliminating it from our bodies. Normally, a healthy colon can handle a certain amount of residue without issues. However, for some individuals, particularly those with certain medical conditions, reducing residue intake becomes essential.

Who Can Benefit from a Low Residue Diet?

A low residue diet is not for everyone; it's tailored to address specific health concerns. This chapter outlines who can benefit from this dietary approach:

1. **Gastrointestinal Disorders:** People with gastrointestinal conditions such as Crohn's disease, ulcerative colitis, diverticulitis, and irritable bowel syndrome (IBS) may

experience flare-ups of symptoms like abdominal pain, diarrhea, and inflammation. For them, minimizing residue can help reduce the irritation and stress on the colon.

2. **Post-Surgery Recovery:** After certain abdominal surgeries, it's common for doctors to recommend a low residue diet to ease the workload on the healing digestive system. This allows the body to recover more comfortably.

3. **Radiation or Chemotherapy:** Cancer

patients undergoing radiation or chemotherapy in the abdominal area may experience digestive issues as side effects. A low residue diet can provide relief from these side effects.

4. **Acute Digestive Symptoms:** Individuals who are experiencing acute digestive symptoms such as diarrhea, cramping, or bloating, regardless of their underlying condition, may temporarily benefit from this diet as it can help reduce the strain on the gut.

What to Expect in This Book

Now that we've established the importance and relevance of a low residue diet, let's discuss what you can expect from this book.

Throughout the chapters to come, we will delve deeper into the nuances of this dietary approach. We'll explore the science behind residue and its impact on the digestive system, outline the potential benefits and risks associated with a low residue diet, and provide practical guidance on how to adopt and sustain this eating plan.

In Chapter 2, we'll explore the concept of residue in more detail and discuss how high-residue foods can affect the digestive system. It's essential to understand the "why" behind this dietary approach, and this chapter will provide the answers.

Chapter 3 will dive into the benefits and risks of a low residue diet. It's crucial to have a balanced perspective on any dietary plan, and we'll discuss both the advantages, such as symptom relief, and the potential drawbacks, including the risk of nutrient deficiencies.

Chapter 4 will serve as a practical guide by providing a comprehensive list of foods to avoid on a low residue diet. Knowing which foods to steer clear of is essential for success in this dietary journey.

Once you've grasped the basics, Chapter 5 will offer guidance on meal planning. We'll share strategies for creating balanced and satisfying meals while adhering to the low residue principles. Sample meal plans catering to different dietary preferences will also be included.

Chapter 6 will tackle nutritional considerations. It's essential to understand how to maintain adequate nutrition while on a low residue diet. We'll discuss potential nutrient deficiencies and the role of supplements in filling those gaps.

Sticking to a specialized diet can be challenging, especially in social situations. Chapter 7 will provide valuable tips for navigating these challenges, handling cravings, and staying on track. Real-life success stories from individuals who have benefited from the diet will serve as inspiration.

Finally, Chapter 8 will address the process of transitioning off the low residue diet when the time is right. We'll provide guidelines for gradually reintroducing higher-residue foods and offer long-term dietary recommendations for maintaining digestive health.

In conclusion, this book is your comprehensive guide to understanding and implementing a low residue diet. Whether you are seeking relief from digestive symptoms or recovering from surgery, our aim is to empower you with knowledge and practical advice to make informed dietary choices and live well with a low residue diet. We encourage you to read on, explore the chapters ahead, and embark on this journey toward better digestive health.

CHAPTER 2

Understanding Residue and Its Impact

In our journey to comprehend the intricacies of a low residue diet, we must start at the very foundation - understanding what residue is and why it matters in the realm of digestion. Chapter 2 delves deeper into this fundamental concept, shedding light on the importance of residue and how it can impact our digestive system.

The Role of Residue in Digestion

At its core, residue is what remains after our body has extracted all the essential nutrients and fluids from the food we consume. Picture it as the aftermath of a grand feast, once the banquet is over, and the essential bits have been collected. This leftover material contains components that our body can't digest or absorb, mainly dietary fiber and waste products.

Now, here's the intriguing part - residue serves an essential role in our digestive process. Fiber, which constitutes a significant portion of residue, is like the broom that sweeps through our intestines, keeping things moving. It adds bulk to our stool, which aids in regular bowel movements and helps prevent constipation. In essence, residue, and particularly dietary fiber, is our digestive system's natural cleaner.

The High-Residue Conundrum

So, if residue is essentially nature's cleaning crew for our digestive system, why would we ever want to reduce it in our diet? Here's where we need to navigate a bit of a paradox.

While dietary fiber is essential for overall health and regular digestion, certain individuals find themselves in situations where high-residue diets can be problematic. This is where a low residue diet comes into play. To understand why this might be necessary, let's explore how high-residue foods can impact our digestive system.

High-Residue Foods and Digestive Challenges

1. **Digestive Disorders:** People with conditions like Crohn's disease, ulcerative colitis, diverticulitis, or

irritable bowel syndrome (IBS) may have inflamed or sensitive intestines. High-residue foods, especially insoluble fiber found in many vegetables and grains, can be abrasive and irritate these already sensitive areas. This irritation can lead to symptoms like abdominal pain, diarrhea, and increased inflammation.

2. **Diverticulosis:** For individuals with diverticulosis, which involves the formation of small pouches in the colon lining, high-residue foods

like nuts, seeds, and popcorn can become trapped in these pouches, causing inflammation and infection (diverticulitis).

3. **Post-Surgery Recovery:** After abdominal surgery, it's common for doctors to recommend a low residue diet. This is because high-residue foods can be difficult to digest, and the digestive system may be temporarily weakened post-surgery. A low residue diet provides a gentler approach to eating during the recovery phase.

4. **Cancer Treatment:** Patients undergoing radiation or chemotherapy in the abdominal area often experience digestive side effects. High-residue foods can exacerbate symptoms like diarrhea, making it necessary to reduce residue intake temporarily.

The Importance of Low Residue Diet

The core principle of a low residue diet is to reduce the workload on the colon. By consuming foods that leave less undigested material behind, the digestive system has less to process, and this can provide several benefits:

1. **Symptom Relief:** For individuals with digestive disorders, adhering to a low residue diet can provide relief from symptoms such as abdominal pain, cramping, diarrhea, and bloating. By minimizing the irritants in the diet, the gut is allowed to calm down.

2. **Colon Healing:** After surgery or during cancer treatment, the digestive system may be in a vulnerable state. A low

residue diet helps protect the healing colon from unnecessary stress, allowing it to recover more comfortably.

3. **Managing Diverticulosis:** For those with diverticulosis, a low residue diet can prevent food particles from getting trapped in the pouches, reducing the risk of inflammation and infection.

4. **Controlled Nutrient Intake:** A low residue diet can also be a tool for managing nutrient intake. In cases where nutrient

absorption needs to be controlled or monitored, such as with certain medical conditions, this dietary approach offers a degree of precision.

Balancing Act: The Low Residue Approach

It's important to note that a low residue diet is not a long-term solution for everyone. In fact, for most individuals with healthy digestive systems, it's not recommended to go on a low residue diet. Dietary fiber, found in high-residue foods, is essential for overall health, regulating cholesterol levels, preventing constipation, and even reducing the risk of chronic diseases like heart disease and type 2 diabetes.

A low residue diet is a specialized approach intended for specific medical situations or temporary relief. It should be implemented under the guidance of a healthcare professional who can assess your individual needs and monitor your progress.

In the next chapters, we'll explore the benefits and potential risks associated with a low residue diet. We'll also provide practical guidance on how to adopt this eating plan, including lists of foods to avoid and meal planning strategies. By the end of this book, you'll be equipped with the knowledge and tools to make informed decisions about whether a low residue diet is right for you and, if so, how to navigate it successfully.

CHAPTER 3

Benefits and Risks of a Low Residue Diet

In our exploration of the low residue diet, we've covered what residue is and why reducing it can be necessary for certain individuals. Now, in Chapter 3, we take a closer look at the balance of benefits and potential risks associated with adopting this dietary approach.

Benefits of a Low Residue Diet:

1. **Symptom Relief:** One of the primary reasons individuals turn to a low residue diet is for symptom relief, especially those with gastrointestinal disorders. Let's delve into some specific conditions where this approach can be immensely beneficial:

    o **Inflammatory Bowel Diseases (IBD):** Conditions like Crohn's disease and ulcerative colitis involve chronic inflammation of the digestive tract. High-residue foods can exacerbate inflammation and symptoms like abdominal pain, diarrhea, and cramping. A low residue diet can provide much-needed relief during flare-ups.

- **Irritable Bowel Syndrome (IBS):** IBS is characterized by digestive symptoms such as bloating, diarrhea, and constipation. High-fiber foods, often considered healthy for most people, can trigger or worsen these symptoms. A low residue diet, tailored to the individual, can help manage IBS symptoms.

o **Diverticulitis:** In diverticulitis, inflammation occurs in the small pouches (diverticula) that can form in the colon. High-residue foods like nuts, seeds, and popcorn can get trapped in these pouches, causing infection and pain. A low residue diet can prevent this by minimizing these irritants.

2. **Post-Surgery Recovery:** Following abdominal surgery, it's common for doctors to recommend a low residue diet. Here's why:

    o **Gentle Healing:** After surgery, the digestive system is in a sensitive state. High-residue foods can be challenging to digest, potentially causing discomfort or complications. A low residue diet eases the digestive workload, allowing the body to heal more comfortably.

3. **Cancer Treatment Support:** Individuals undergoing radiation or chemotherapy in the abdominal area often experience digestive side effects. High-residue foods can exacerbate symptoms like diarrhea, which can be particularly distressing during cancer treatment. A

low residue diet can provide relief from these side effects.

4. **Controlled Nutrient Intake:** In certain medical conditions, precise control over nutrient intake is necessary. A low residue diet can be a tool for managing this. By reducing residue, it's possible to fine-tune nutrient absorption, which may be crucial in specific medical contexts.

Potential Risks and Drawbacks of a Low Residue Diet:

While a low residue diet can offer significant benefits, it's not without potential risks and drawbacks. It's crucial to consider these factors before adopting this dietary approach:

1. **Nutrient Deficiencies:** By limiting high-fiber foods, a low residue diet can potentially lead to nutrient deficiencies. Fiber is essential for overall health, regulating cholesterol levels, preventing constipation, and supporting a healthy gut microbiome. When significantly reducing fiber

intake, individuals may miss out on these benefits.

- o **Counteraction:** To mitigate this risk, healthcare professionals often recommend supplements and monitoring to ensure that necessary nutrients are still being provided. Multivitamins and mineral supplements can help bridge nutritional gaps.

2. **Long-Term Health:** For individuals without specific

medical conditions, a long-term low residue diet can have negative health implications. Without an adequate intake of fiber-rich foods, there's an increased risk of chronic diseases such as heart disease, type 2 diabetes, and certain types of cancer.

- **Balanced Approach:** If you don't have a medical need for a low residue diet, it's essential to focus on a balanced and varied diet that includes fiber-rich foods, such as fruits, vegetables, whole grains, and legumes. These foods offer a multitude of health benefits beyond digestion.

3. **Digestive Adaptation:** Over time, the digestive system can adapt to the foods we consume regularly. If a low residue diet is maintained for an extended period, the digestive tract may become less accustomed to processing high-fiber foods. This can make transitioning back to a

regular diet more challenging.

- **Guided Transition:** It's vital to work closely with a healthcare provider when transitioning off a low residue diet to ensure a gradual and smooth return to a more typical eating plan.

The Importance of Individualization:

One crucial aspect to emphasize is that the decision to adopt a low residue diet should be highly individualized. It's not a one-size-fits-all approach. Each person's dietary needs and health conditions vary, and thus, the benefits and risks will differ.

The guidance of a healthcare professional is paramount. If you are considering a low residue diet, it's essential to consult with a doctor or registered dietitian who can assess your specific health situation and provide personalized recommendations.

Monitoring and Regular Evaluation:

Whether you're following a low residue diet for symptom relief or as part of a medical treatment plan, regular monitoring and evaluation are crucial. Your healthcare provider can track your progress, assess your nutritional status, and make necessary adjustments to ensure your dietary needs are being met while minimizing potential risks.

Conclusion: Balancing Act and Informed Decisions

In Chapter 3, we've explored the intricate balance between the benefits and potential risks of a low residue diet. It's not a dietary approach to be taken lightly; rather, it's a tool to be used strategically in specific medical contexts.

The key takeaway is the importance of informed decisions. Before embarking on a low residue diet, carefully consider your unique health situation, and seek guidance from healthcare professionals who can provide expert advice and ongoing support.

As we move forward in this book, we'll provide more practical guidance on adopting and maintaining a low residue diet, including comprehensive lists of foods to avoid, meal planning strategies, and tips for navigating social situations. Armed with knowledge and personalized guidance, you can make the right choices for your digestive health.

CHAPTER 4

Foods to Avoid on a Low Residue Diet

In our journey to understand the low residue diet, we've explored the significance of residue, its impact on the digestive system, and the balance of benefits and risks. Now, in Chapter 4, we'll dive into practical details by providing a comprehensive list of foods to avoid when following this dietary approach.

The core principle of a low residue diet is to minimize dietary residue, particularly indigestible components like fiber. To achieve this, individuals are advised to restrict or completely avoid certain types of foods. Here's a detailed breakdown of these foods:

High-Fiber Vegetables:

1. **Raw Vegetables:** Raw vegetables are often rich in fiber and can be difficult to digest. These include salads, raw broccoli, cauliflower, and bell peppers.

2. **Cruciferous Vegetables:** Vegetables like cabbage, Brussels sprouts, and kale

are not recommended due to
their high fiber content.

3. **Corn:** Corn kernels are high in fiber and should be avoided in their whole form.

4. **Beans and Legumes:** Beans, lentils, and chickpeas are excellent sources of fiber but are generally not suitable for a low residue diet.

High-Fiber Fruits: 5. **Berries:** Raspberries, blackberries, strawberries, and similar fruits are packed with fiber and should be avoided.

6. **Dried Fruits:** Prunes, raisins, and other dried

fruits are concentrated sources of fiber and can be challenging to digest.

7. **Citrus Fruits:** Oranges, grapefruits, and other citrus fruits are high in fiber and may irritate the digestive system.

8. **Fruit Skins:** The skins of fruits, such as apples, pears, and grapes, are particularly fibrous and should be peeled before consumption.

Whole Grains: 9. **Whole Wheat Products:** Bread, pasta, and other products made from whole wheat flour are high in fiber and should be avoided.

10. **Whole Grain Cereals:** Cereals like bran flakes, whole grain oats, and granola are rich in fiber and are not suitable for a low residue diet.

11. **Brown Rice:** Unlike white rice, brown rice contains the bran layer, which is high in fiber.

12. **Whole Grain Crackers:** Snack items like whole grain crackers and rice cakes are fiber-rich and should be limited.

Nuts and Seeds: 13. **Nuts:** Almonds, peanuts, walnuts, and other nuts are dense sources of fiber and are typically not included in a low residue diet.

14.**Seeds:** Flaxseeds, chia seeds, pumpkin seeds, and similar seeds are high in fiber and should be avoided.

High-Residue Proteins: 15. **Tough Meat and Poultry:** Tough cuts of meat and poultry can be difficult to digest. These include steak, roast beef, and skin-on poultry.

16. **Processed Meats:** Highly processed meats like sausages, hot dogs, and deli meats often contain added fillers and fiber-rich ingredients.

Miscellaneous High-Residue Foods: 17. **Popcorn:** The hulls of popcorn kernels are indigestible and can irritate the digestive tract.

18. **Tough, Chewy Foods:** Foods that are tough or chewy, like beef jerky or tough cuts of meat, should be avoided.

19. **Coconut:** Coconut, whether fresh or dried, is relatively

high in fiber and should be limited.

20.   **Mushrooms:** While they are not particularly high in fiber, mushrooms can be challenging to digest and are typically avoided on a low residue diet.

Beverages and Liquids: 21. **Alcohol:** Alcoholic beverages can irritate the digestive system and should be consumed in moderation or avoided.

22.   **Carbonated Drinks:** Carbonated beverages can contribute to gas and

discomfort and are best avoided.

23.   **Fruit Juices:** Fruit juices, especially those high in pulp, can be rich in fiber and should be limited.

Condiments and Seasonings:
24. **Hot Peppers and Spicy Foods:** Spicy foods can irritate the digestive tract and may need to be avoided, depending on individual tolerance.

25.   **High-Fiber Sauces:** Sauces and condiments that contain chunks of vegetables or herbs should be used sparingly.

Food Additives and Supplements: 26. Fiber Supplements: Products like psyllium husk or metamucil, which are designed to increase fiber intake, should be avoided on a low residue diet.

27. **Artificial Sweeteners:** Some artificial sweeteners, like sorbitol and mannitol, can have a laxative effect and may need to be limited.

Tips for Reading Food Labels:

Navigating a low residue diet also involves becoming skilled at reading food labels. Here are some tips for identifying high-residue foods when shopping:

- **Check the Fiber Content:** Pay close attention to the dietary fiber content listed on the Nutrition Facts label. Foods with high fiber content should be avoided or limited.

- **Look for Whole Grains:** Whole grains often have a denser texture and higher fiber content. Opt for refined grains instead.

- **Inspect Ingredient Lists:** Scan the ingredient list for foods that contain high-residue ingredients like whole wheat, bran, nuts, seeds, or dried fruits.

Customization: Tailoring the Diet to Individual Needs:

It's crucial to remember that the severity of dietary restrictions on a low residue diet can vary based on an individual's health condition and tolerance. Some individuals may be able to tolerate small amounts of certain high-residue foods, while others may need to be more strict in their avoidance.

Conclusion: Building a Low Residue Diet

Chapter 4 has provided a detailed list of foods to avoid on a low residue diet. These restrictions are designed to minimize the amount of undigested material in the digestive tract, providing relief for individuals with specific medical conditions or during certain treatment phases.

However, it's essential to approach this dietary plan under the guidance of a healthcare professional, as individual needs and tolerances can vary widely. Additionally, in Chapter 5, we'll delve into the practical aspects of building a low residue diet, offering strategies for meal planning, cooking techniques, and sample meal plans to help you navigate this dietary approach effectively while ensuring balanced nutrition.

CHAPTER 5

Low Residue Diet Meal Planning

In Chapter 4, we discussed the foods to avoid on a low residue diet to minimize undigested material in the digestive tract. Now, in Chapter 5, we dive into the practical side of adopting this dietary approach, focusing on low residue diet meal planning.

Meal planning is a critical component of any diet, but it becomes even more important when you're following a specialized eating plan like the low residue diet. Proper planning ensures you get the necessary nutrients while avoiding high-residue foods. Let's explore some essential aspects of meal planning for a low residue diet.

1. Understanding Portion Sizes:

One of the first things to consider is portion sizes. Since you'll be avoiding many high-fiber foods, it's important to maintain an appropriate calorie intake and get essential nutrients. Consider consulting a registered dietitian who can help you determine the right portion sizes based on your specific dietary needs and health goals.

2. Balancing Macronutrients:

A well-balanced low residue diet should include an appropriate balance of macronutrients: carbohydrates, protein, and fats. Here's how to do that:

- **Carbohydrates:** Opt for refined grains and starches like white rice, white bread, and pasta. These are lower in fiber and gentler on the digestive system.

Incorporate them into your meals to provide energy.

- **Protein:** Choose lean protein sources such as skinless poultry, fish, eggs, and well-cooked, tender meat. These protein sources are easier to digest and less likely to irritate the digestive tract.

- **Fats:** Include sources of healthy fats like avocados, olive oil, and nut butters in your diet. Fats provide essential nutrients and can add flavor and variety to your meals.

3. Food Texture and Preparation:

The texture and preparation of foods can make a significant difference when you're on a low residue diet. Here are some tips:

- **Cooking Techniques:** Focus on cooking methods that make foods softer and easier to digest, such as boiling, poaching, steaming, and baking. These methods help break down the fibers and make food more tender.

- **Blending and Pureeing:** In some cases, blending or pureeing foods can be beneficial, especially if you have difficulty chewing or swallowing. This can be particularly useful for fruits, vegetables, and legumes.

- **Avoid Overcooking:** While it's essential to make foods tender, avoid overcooking, which can make them mushy and less appetizing. Aim for a balance between soft and palatable textures.

4. Meal Timing:

Consider the timing of your meals and snacks. Eating smaller, more frequent meals throughout the day can be easier on your digestive system than having three large meals. This approach can also help prevent overeating and manage symptoms.

5. Sample Low Residue Diet Meal Plans:

Here are two sample meal plans to give you a sense of how to structure your daily meals on a low residue diet. Keep in mind that individual dietary needs and preferences may vary, so these are just examples:

Sample Meal Plan 1:

Breakfast:

- Scrambled eggs with a small amount of cheese
- White toast (no butter or jam)
- Sliced, peeled apples

Snack:

- Greek yogurt (choose a low-fiber variety)
- Clear fruit juice (strained)

Lunch:

- Grilled chicken breast (soft and tender)
- White rice
- Cooked carrots (mashed or pureed)
- Water or herbal tea

Snack:

- Banana (ripe)
- Cottage cheese (low-fat)

Dinner:

- Baked salmon (flaky and tender)
- Mashed potatoes (without skins)
- Steamed zucchini (soft and well-cooked)
- Lemon water

Sample Meal Plan 2:

Breakfast:

- Cream of wheat or rice cereal (smooth consistency)
- Poached egg
- Applesauce (no skins)

Snack:

- Smooth peanut butter on white bread (no crust)
- Sliced, ripe melon

Lunch:

- Turkey sandwich on white bread (no lettuce or tomato)
- Low-residue potato salad
- Clear soup (strained broth)

Snack:

- Low-fiber crackers

- Hummus (small portion)

Dinner:

- Baked tilapia (flaky and mild)

- Mashed sweet potatoes (no skins)

- Cooked spinach (well-cooked and pureed)

- Water with lemon

6. Food Substitutions:

One of the keys to successful meal planning on a low residue diet is finding suitable substitutions for high-residue ingredients. Here are some common substitutions to consider:

- **White Rice Instead of Brown Rice:** Choose white rice over brown rice, as it's lower in fiber and easier to digest.

- **White Bread Over Whole Wheat:** Opt for white bread instead of whole wheat bread to reduce fiber intake.

- **Peeled and Cooked Vegetables:** If you want to include vegetables, choose well-cooked, peeled, and pureed options, like mashed potatoes or carrot puree.

- **Tender Cuts of Meat:** Select lean and tender cuts of meat or poultry that are easier to chew and digest.

- **Cooked Fruits:** If you'd like to include fruit, consider cooking it to soften the texture. Applesauce and cooked pears are good options.

7. Stay Hydrated:

Maintaining proper hydration is essential, especially if you have diarrhea or are prone to it. Drinking plenty of water is crucial. You can also enjoy clear fluids like herbal teas, strained broths, and clear juices.

8. Consult with a Dietitian:

A registered dietitian can be an invaluable resource when planning your low residue diet. They can tailor your meal plans to meet your specific dietary needs and ensure that you're getting the essential nutrients your body requires.

Conclusion: The Art of Low Residue Meal Planning

Chapter 5 has delved into the practical side of adopting a low residue diet through meal planning. Balancing macronutrients, choosing suitable food textures, and making wise substitutions are key aspects to consider. Remember that meal planning should be personalized to your unique dietary needs and preferences.

As we move forward in this book, we'll continue to provide practical guidance and support for your low residue diet journey. In Chapter 6, we'll explore nutritional considerations, including potential nutrient deficiencies and the role of supplements in maintaining balanced nutrition while on this dietary approach.

CHAPTER 6

Nutritional Considerations on a Low Residue Diet

In the previous chapters, we've covered the fundamentals of a low residue diet, its benefits and risks, foods to avoid, and practical meal planning. Now, in Chapter 6, we'll delve into important nutritional considerations. Maintaining proper nutrition while on this dietary approach is paramount for overall health and well-being.

A low residue diet, by design, restricts the intake of high-fiber foods, which can increase the risk of nutrient deficiencies if not managed thoughtfully. In this chapter, we'll explore:

1. **Nutrient Deficiencies on a Low Residue Diet**
2. **The Role of Supplements**
3. **Monitoring Nutritional Intake**

Nutrient Deficiencies on a Low Residue Diet:

When you limit high-fiber foods, you inevitably reduce your intake of essential nutrients. Here are some nutrients that may be at risk of deficiency on a low residue diet and their significance for health:

1. Fiber:

- **Role:** Fiber plays a crucial role in maintaining regular bowel movements, preventing constipation, and supporting a healthy gut microbiome.

- **Deficiency Risk:** Since a low residue diet restricts fiber intake, you won't get the full benefits of this nutrient. However, for some individuals with specific medical conditions, reducing fiber is necessary for symptom management.

2. Vitamins and Minerals:

- **Role:** Various vitamins and minerals are essential for overall health, including immune function, energy metabolism, and bone health.

- **Deficiency Risk:** Depending on your dietary choices within the low residue diet, you may be at risk of deficiencies in vitamins like vitamin C, vitamin K, and folic acid, as well as minerals such as potassium and magnesium. These nutrients are often found in fruits, vegetables, and whole grains, which are restricted on this diet.

3. Protein:

- **Role:** Protein is crucial for tissue repair, immune function, and maintaining muscle mass.

- **Deficiency Risk:** While a low residue diet allows for lean protein sources like poultry and fish, if not balanced properly, it can still pose a risk of inadequate protein intake.

4. Healthy Fats:

- **Role:** Healthy fats, such as those found in avocados and olive oil, provide essential fatty acids and support overall health.

- **Deficiency Risk:** On a low residue diet, fats can be a valuable source of calories and nutrients. Ensuring an adequate intake of healthy fats is essential for overall well-being.

5. Calcium and Vitamin D:

- **Role:** Calcium and vitamin D are essential for bone health.

- **Deficiency Risk:** Dairy products, which are rich sources of calcium and vitamin D, are often limited on a low residue diet. Ensuring you get enough of these nutrients may require careful planning or supplementation.

The Role of Supplements:

Supplements can play a vital role in filling the nutrient gaps that may arise on a low residue diet. Here are some supplements to consider, but it's essential to consult with a healthcare provider or registered dietitian before starting any supplementation:

1. Multivitamins and Minerals:

- **Role:** A multivitamin and mineral supplement can help cover a broad range of nutrient needs. Look for one that is appropriate for your age, gender, and specific dietary restrictions.

- **Consideration:** Be cautious not to overdo it with supplements, as excessive intake of certain vitamins and minerals can be harmful. Follow your healthcare provider's guidance regarding dosages.

2. Fiber Supplements:

- **Role:** In some cases, healthcare providers may recommend a fiber supplement, especially for individuals who need to manage diarrhea or maintain regular bowel movements. These supplements are generally soluble fibers, which are gentler on the digestive system.

- **Consideration:** Fiber supplements should only be used under medical supervision, as they can exacerbate symptoms in some individuals.

3. Calcium and Vitamin D:

- **Role:** If your dietary calcium and vitamin D intake is limited due to a low residue diet, your healthcare provider may recommend supplements to support bone health.

- **Consideration:** Ensure that you are taking these supplements in the right doses and in conjunction with your dietary intake. Excessive intake of calcium and vitamin D can have adverse effects.

Monitoring Nutritional Intake:

Maintaining balanced nutrition on a low residue diet requires vigilance and careful tracking. Here are some steps to monitor your nutritional intake effectively:

1. Keep a Food Diary:

- **Purpose:** A food diary can help you track what you eat

and identify any potential deficiencies.

- **What to Record:** Note the foods you consume, portion sizes, and any supplements you take. Be as detailed as possible.

2. Regularly Review with a Healthcare Provider:

- **Purpose:** Regular check-ins with your healthcare provider or registered dietitian are essential for evaluating your nutritional status and making any necessary adjustments.

- **Frequency:** The frequency of these check-ins may vary based on your individual health needs, but aim for regular follow-ups, especially when first implementing the diet.

3. Be Mindful of Food Choices:

- **Purpose:** Be conscious of the nutrient content of the foods you choose to include in your low residue diet.

- **Strategies:** Opt for nutrient-dense foods when possible. For example, choose lean proteins, incorporate healthy fats, and select low-residue fruits and vegetables like peeled and cooked options.

## 4.	Explore	Cooking Techniques:

- **Purpose:**	Cooking techniques can impact the nutrient content and digestibility of foods.
- **Techniques:** Experiment with different cooking methods to make foods more tender and easier to digest, such as boiling, poaching, and steaming.

5. Adjust Your Diet as Needed:

- **Purpose:** If you identify nutrient deficiencies or symptoms related to your diet, be prepared to adjust your dietary plan.

- **Consultation:** Always consult with a healthcare provider or registered dietitian before making significant dietary changes. They can provide guidance on how to address specific deficiencies.

Conclusion: Maintaining Nutrition on a Low Residue Diet

Chapter 6 has shed light on the nutritional considerations of a low residue diet. While this dietary approach restricts certain high-fiber foods, careful planning and, if necessary, supplementation can help ensure you're getting the essential nutrients your body needs.

Balancing macronutrients, monitoring micronutrients, and collaborating with healthcare professionals are key to maintaining your overall health and well-being while following a low residue diet. In Chapter 7, we'll address practical strategies for staying on track and coping with challenges, including tips for navigating social situations and managing cravings, to help you succeed in your dietary journey.

CHAPTER 7

Practical Strategies for Success on a Low Residue Diet

In the preceding chapters, we've delved into the intricacies of a low residue diet, from understanding what it is to meal planning and nutritional considerations. Now, in Chapter 7, we'll explore practical strategies to help you succeed in implementing and maintaining this dietary approach.

A low residue diet can present unique challenges, both in terms of dietary restrictions and lifestyle adjustments. However, armed with knowledge and some practical strategies, you can navigate these challenges with confidence.

1. Navigating Social Situations:

Eating is often a social activity, and adhering to a special diet can sometimes be challenging in social settings. Here are some tips for navigating social situations while on a low residue diet:

- **Communicate:** Inform friends and family about

your dietary restrictions so they can accommodate your needs when planning gatherings or meals.

- **Offer to Contribute:** When attending potlucks or gatherings, offer to bring a dish that fits within your dietary restrictions. This ensures you have a safe and enjoyable option to eat.

- **Choose Restaurants Wisely:** When dining out, research restaurant menus in advance or call ahead to inquire about low residue options. Many restaurants are willing to accommodate dietary needs.

- **Stay Hydrated:** If alcohol is being served, limit your consumption as it can irritate the digestive tract. Instead, opt for non-alcoholic beverages like sparkling water or herbal tea.

- **Be Mindful of Portions:** While socializing, it's easy to overindulge. Be mindful of portion sizes to prevent discomfort.

2. Managing Cravings:

Cravings for high-residue foods can be challenging to overcome on a low residue diet. Here's how to manage cravings effectively:

- **Plan Treats Mindfully:** It's okay to indulge occasionally, but plan these indulgences mindfully. Allow yourself small portions of your favorite high-residue treats when you truly crave them.

- **Seek Alternatives:** Look for low residue alternatives that satisfy your cravings. For example, if you're craving potato chips, try baked or thinly sliced and baked potatoes as a substitute.

- **Stay Occupied:** Distractions like hobbies or physical activities can help take your mind off cravings. Sometimes, cravings are more about boredom than actual hunger.

- **Stay Hydrated:** Thirst can often masquerade as hunger or cravings. Drinking water or herbal tea can help curb cravings.

3. Meal Preparation and Planning:

Effective meal planning is key to success on a low residue diet. Here are some strategies to make meal preparation easier and more efficient:

- **Batch Cooking:** Prepare larger quantities of low residue-friendly foods and freeze them in individual portions. This saves time on busy days when you may not feel like cooking.

- **Meal Prep:** Spend some time each week preparing ingredients like peeled and cooked vegetables, lean proteins, and low-fiber grains. Having these components ready makes it easier to assemble meals quickly.

- **Use Appliances:** Invest in kitchen appliances like a slow cooker or instant pot. These can help you prepare tender and easily digestible meals with minimal effort.

- **Plan Ahead:** Plan your meals for the week in advance. This allows you to create a shopping list and ensure you have the necessary ingredients on hand.

4. Handling Digestive Symptoms:

Digestive symptoms can be a concern when following a low residue diet. Here's how to manage them effectively:

- **Keep a Symptom Journal:** Maintain a journal to track your symptoms, including what you ate and any reactions you experienced. This can help identify trigger foods or patterns.

- **Stay Hydrated:** Proper hydration is essential, especially if you have diarrhea. Dehydration can exacerbate symptoms. Drink plenty of water throughout the day.

- **Consider Medication:** If your symptoms are severe or persistent, discuss medication options with your healthcare provider. They can recommend over-the-counter or prescription medications to help manage symptoms.

- **Consult a Dietitian:** If you're struggling with symptoms, consult with a registered dietitian who can offer personalized advice and meal planning strategies to alleviate discomfort.

5. Adapting to Lifestyle Changes:

A low residue diet may require some lifestyle adjustments. Here are ways to adapt effectively:

- **Exercise Wisely:** Regular physical activity is important, but be mindful of the timing. Strenuous exercise immediately after eating can exacerbate digestive discomfort. Allow time for digestion before engaging in intense workouts.

- **Stress Management:** Stress can affect digestive health. Practice stress-reduction techniques like meditation, deep breathing, or yoga to help manage symptoms.

- **Travel Planning:** When traveling, plan your meals carefully. Research restaurants at your destination that offer low residue options, and consider packing suitable snacks for the journey.

- **Medication Management:** If you're taking medications, ensure they align with your dietary restrictions. Some medications may need to be taken with food or specific types of foods.

6. Seek Support:

Living with dietary restrictions can be challenging, and you don't have to do it alone. Seek support from friends, family, or online communities of individuals with similar dietary needs. Sharing experiences and tips can be invaluable.

7. Reintroducing High-Residue Foods:

In some cases, a low residue diet is temporary, and you may need to reintroduce high-residue foods gradually. Here's how to approach this:

- **Consult Your Healthcare Provider:** Before reintroducing high-residue foods, consult with your healthcare provider or dietitian. They can provide guidance on the best way to do this based on your specific health needs.

- **Take It Slow:** Start by introducing small amounts of high-residue foods and monitor your body's response. Gradually increase the amounts as tolerated.

- **Pay Attention to Symptoms:** Be mindful of any symptoms or discomfort that arise when reintroducing these foods. This information can guide your dietary choices.

Conclusion: Thriving on a Low Residue Diet

Chapter 7 has explored practical strategies to help you succeed on a low residue diet. From navigating social situations and managing cravings to adapting to lifestyle changes and reintroducing high-residue foods, these strategies are designed to empower you to thrive within the constraints of this dietary approach.

Remember that every person's experience with a low residue diet is unique, and it may take time to find the balance that works best for you. With patience, support, and thoughtful planning, you can successfully manage your dietary needs while maintaining your overall health and well-being.

CHAPTER 8

Long-Term Management and Beyond: Life After a Low Residue Diet

In this final chapter, we'll explore the long-term management of a low residue diet and what life looks like beyond this dietary approach. While the low residue diet serves specific medical purposes, many individuals wonder what happens next. What dietary options are available, and how can you transition back to a more typical eating pattern without compromising your health?

1. Transitioning from a Low Residue Diet:

Transitioning from a low residue diet back to a regular diet is a significant milestone. However, this process should be gradual and guided by healthcare professionals. Here's how to navigate this transition:

- **Consult Your Healthcare Provider:** Before making any dietary changes, consult with your healthcare provider or dietitian. They can assess your health status and provide personalized recommendations for transitioning back to a regular diet.

- **Gradual Reintroduction:** High-residue foods should be reintroduced slowly and in small quantities. Pay close attention to how your body responds, as individual tolerance varies.

- **Monitoring Symptoms:** Continue to track your symptoms and dietary choices during the transition period. This information can guide adjustments and ensure a smooth transition.

- **Balanced Diet:** As you reintroduce high-residue foods, focus on achieving a balanced diet that includes a variety of fruits, vegetables, whole grains, lean proteins, and healthy fats. This balanced approach is crucial for long-term health.

2. Maintaining Digestive Health:

After transitioning from a low residue diet, maintaining digestive health becomes a top priority. Here are some key considerations:

- **Fiber Intake:** Gradually increase your fiber intake by incorporating more fruits, vegetables, whole grains, and legumes into your diet. Aim for the recommended daily amount of fiber, but do so gradually to minimize digestive discomfort.

- **Hydration:** Continue to stay well-hydrated, as adequate fluid intake supports healthy digestion and regular bowel movements.

- **Probiotics:** Probiotic-rich foods like yogurt and kefir, or probiotic supplements, can help promote a healthy gut microbiome. Consult your healthcare provider for guidance on incorporating probiotics into your diet.

- **Regular Exercise:** Physical activity supports digestive health by promoting regular bowel movements. Incorporate regular exercise into your routine to maintain digestive well-being.

3. Dietary Flexibility and Variety:

While a low residue diet restricts many high-fiber foods, it's essential to embrace dietary flexibility and variety once you've transitioned. Here's how:

- **Explore New Foods:** Use this opportunity to explore a wider range of foods and cuisines. Trying new foods can make your meals more exciting and nutritious.
- **Mindful Eating:** Practice mindful eating, which involves savoring and enjoying your food. This can help you better appreciate the flavors and textures of different foods.

- **Balanced Diet:** Strive for a balanced diet that includes all food groups. Incorporate lean proteins, whole grains, colorful fruits and vegetables, and healthy fats into your meals.

4. Ongoing Medical Management:

Certain medical conditions, such as Crohn's disease, ulcerative colitis, or diverticulitis, may require ongoing medical management even after transitioning from a low residue diet. Here's what to consider:

- **Medications:** Continue to take any prescribed medications as directed by your healthcare provider. These medications play a crucial role in managing your condition.

- **Regular Check-Ups:** Schedule regular check-ups with your healthcare provider to monitor your health and discuss any concerns or changes in your condition.

- **Dietary Modifications:** Depending on your condition, you may need to make specific dietary modifications to manage symptoms or prevent flare-ups. Consult your healthcare provider or a registered dietitian for guidance.

5. Meal Planning for Life:

Regardless of your dietary history, meal planning remains an important aspect of maintaining a healthy lifestyle. Here are some tips for successful meal planning:

- **Plan Ahead:** Take time each week to plan your meals and create a shopping list. Planning ahead helps you make healthier choices and reduce food waste.

- **Variety:** Aim for variety in your meals by incorporating different foods from all food groups. This ensures you get a wide range of nutrients.

- **Portion Control:** Be mindful of portion sizes to avoid overeating. Use smaller plates and utensils to help with portion control.

- **Cook at Home:** Whenever possible, cook meals at home, where you have control over the ingredients and preparation methods.

6. Seeking Support and Education:

Living with a chronic digestive condition can be challenging, both physically and emotionally. Seeking support and education can make a significant difference in your overall well-being:

- **Support Groups:** Consider joining a support group for individuals with similar digestive conditions. Sharing experiences and advice can provide emotional support and valuable insights.

- **Continued Learning:** Stay informed about your specific

condition and treatment options. Knowledge empowers you to make informed decisions about your health.

- **Psychological Support:** If you experience emotional challenges related to your condition, consider seeking support from a therapist or counselor who specializes in chronic illness.

7. The Role of a Registered Dietitian:

A registered dietitian can be a valuable resource throughout your journey, from managing a low residue diet to transitioning back to a regular diet and beyond. They can provide personalized guidance, meal planning strategies, and ongoing support to help you achieve and maintain optimal digestive health.

Conclusion: Embracing a Healthy Future

Chapter 8 has explored life after a low residue diet, emphasizing the importance of gradual transitions, ongoing digestive health maintenance, and the role of support and education. It's crucial to remember that managing a chronic digestive condition is a lifelong journey that requires patience, flexibility, and a proactive approach to health.

As you move forward, continue to collaborate closely with your healthcare provider and registered dietitian to ensure you're making the best choices for your specific health needs. By embracing a balanced diet, maintaining digestive health, seeking support, and staying informed, you can look forward to a healthy future beyond the limitations of a low residue diet.

CONCLUSION

In conclusion, the journey through the chapters of this book on the low residue diet has been a comprehensive exploration of a dietary approach that serves a specific purpose in managing digestive conditions. From understanding the fundamentals and risks to mastering meal planning, nutritional considerations, practical strategies, and life after the diet, we've covered a wide spectrum of knowledge and guidance.

The low residue diet is not just about dietary restrictions; it's a pathway to better managing specific medical conditions, reducing symptoms, and improving overall well-being. It highlights the significance of balance, flexibility, and mindful choices when it comes to what we eat and how it affects our bodies.

Whether you or someone you know is following this diet for medical reasons or out of curiosity, the key takeaway is that it's a tool to be used under the guidance of healthcare professionals. It's a stepping stone towards better digestive health, but it's not the final destination. Life after a low residue diet involves careful transitions, ongoing monitoring, and a commitment to maintaining overall health.

Remember that you are not alone in this journey. Seek support from healthcare providers, registered dietitians, support groups, and your own network of friends and family. Embrace the knowledge you've gained and the practical strategies you've learned to navigate the challenges of dietary restrictions and to make informed choices for a healthier future.

Ultimately, this book serves as a resource, a guide, and a source of empowerment. Whether you're just starting the low residue diet, in the midst of it, or moving beyond it, know that your health and well-being are worth the effort, the learning, and the journey. Here's to your continued path towards a healthier, happier, and more resilient digestive future.